DR. BARBARA'S SIMPLE CURE FOR TYPE 2 DIABETES

Discover Dr. Barbara's natural remedies: reverse type 2 diabetes naturally with holistic healing method and embrace a diabetes-free life

I0781598

Emily Kent

Table of Contents

COPYRIGHT © 2023

CHAPTER ONE

Understanding Type 2 Diabetes: Causes, Symptoms, and Complications

Type 2 diabetes is a chronic metabolic disorder characterized by high blood sugar levels, insulin resistance, and relative insulin deficiency. It is the most common form of diabetes, comprising approximately 90% of all diagnosed cases worldwide. Understanding the causes, symptoms, and potential complications of type 2 diabetes is crucial for effective management and prevention.

Causes of Type 2 Diabetes:

Type 2 diabetes develops when the body becomes resistant to insulin or when the pancreas fails to produce enough insulin to maintain normal blood sugar levels. Several factors contribute to the development of insulin resistance and subsequent type 2 diabetes:

1. **Genetic Predisposition:** Genetics plays a significant role in the development of type 2 diabetes. Individuals with a family history of the disease are at a higher risk of developing it themselves.

2. **Lifestyle Factors:** Sedentary lifestyle, poor dietary habits, and obesity are major contributors to the development of

type 2 diabetes. Excess body weight, especially around the abdomen, increases insulin resistance.

3. **Insulin Resistance:** Insulin resistance occurs when cells in the body become less responsive to the effects of insulin. This forces the pancreas to produce more insulin to compensate, eventually leading to impaired insulin secretion.

4. **Age and Ethnicity:** Advancing age is a risk factor for type 2 diabetes, with incidence increasing significantly after the age of 45. Certain ethnic groups, such as African Americans, Hispanic/Latino Americans, and Native Americans, are also at higher risk.

5. **Medical Conditions:** Certain medical conditions, such as polycystic ovary syndrome (PCOS), prediabetes, and gestational diabetes during pregnancy, increase the risk of developing type 2 diabetes.

Symptoms of Type 2 Diabetes:

Type 2 diabetes often develops gradually, and symptoms may not be immediately apparent. Some individuals may not experience any symptoms initially, leading to delayed diagnosis. Common symptoms of type 2 diabetes include:

1. **Increased Thirst and Urination:** Excess sugar in the blood leads to increased thirst (polydipsia) and frequent urination (polyuria) as the body tries to eliminate the excess glucose.

2. **Fatigue:** Despite increased calorie intake, individuals with type 2 diabetes may experience fatigue and weakness due to the body's inability to effectively utilize glucose for energy.

3. **Weight Changes:** Unexplained weight loss or gain may occur in individuals with type 2 diabetes, often due to fluctuations in fluid levels and changes in metabolism.

4. **Blurred Vision:** High blood sugar levels can cause temporary changes in the shape of the lens in the eye, leading to blurred vision or difficulty focusing.

5. **Slow Healing:** Wounds and infections may take longer to heal in individuals with type 2 diabetes due to impaired circulation and compromised immune function.

6. **Numbness and Tingling:** Peripheral neuropathy, characterized by numbness, tingling, or pain in the hands and feet, is a common complication of long-term uncontrolled diabetes.

Complications of Type 2 Diabetes:

Untreated or poorly managed type 2 diabetes can lead to a wide range of complications affecting various organs and systems in the body:

1. **Cardiovascular Complications:** Type 2 diabetes significantly increases the risk of cardiovascular diseases, such as heart attack, stroke, and peripheral artery disease, due to the

damaging effects of high blood sugar levels on blood vessels and the heart.

2. **Neuropathy:** Chronic high blood sugar levels can damage the nerves throughout the body, leading to neuropathy. Peripheral neuropathy affects the nerves in the extremities, causing pain, numbness, and tingling, while autonomic neuropathy affects the nerves that control involuntary bodily functions, leading to digestive issues, bladder problems, and sexual dysfunction.

3. **Nephropathy:** Diabetes is a leading cause of kidney disease (nephropathy), characterized by impaired kidney function and eventual kidney failure. Persistent high blood sugar levels can damage the small blood vessels in the kidneys, leading to proteinuria (protein in the urine) and decreased kidney function.

4. **Retinopathy:** Diabetes can damage the blood vessels in the retina (diabetic retinopathy), leading to vision impairment and blindness if left untreated. Early detection and intervention are crucial to prevent vision loss.

5. **Foot Complications:** Peripheral neuropathy and poor circulation increase the risk of foot problems in individuals with type 2 diabetes. Untreated foot ulcers can lead to serious infections and, in severe cases, amputation.

6. **Skin Conditions:** Diabetes increases the risk of various skin conditions, including bacterial and fungal infections, itching, and dry skin. Poorly controlled blood sugar levels create an environment conducive to bacterial and fungal growth.

7. **Mental Health Issues:** Living with a chronic condition like type 2 diabetes can take a toll on mental health, leading to depression, anxiety, and diabetes distress. It's essential for individuals with diabetes to prioritize their mental well-being and seek support when needed.

In conclusion, type 2 diabetes is a complex metabolic disorder with multifactorial causes, diverse symptoms, and potential complications affecting various organ systems. Early diagnosis, lifestyle modifications, and appropriate medical management are essential for preventing and minimizing the impact of type 2 diabetes on overall health and quality of life. Regular monitoring, adherence to treatment plans, and ongoing support from healthcare professionals are critical components of comprehensive diabetes care.

CHAPTER TWO

The Role of Lifestyle Factors in Managing Type 2 Diabetes

Type 2 diabetes is a chronic condition that is largely influenced by lifestyle factors. While genetic predisposition plays a role in its development, lifestyle choices such as diet, physical activity, and weight management are key determinants in its management and prevention. Adopting a healthy lifestyle can significantly improve blood sugar control, reduce the risk of complications, and enhance overall well-being for individuals with type 2 diabetes. In this discussion, we'll delve into the crucial role of lifestyle factors in managing type 2 diabetes and explore effective strategies for implementing positive changes.

Dietary Choices:

One of the cornerstones of managing type 2 diabetes is maintaining a balanced and nutritious diet. Dietary choices directly impact blood sugar levels, insulin sensitivity, and overall health. Here are some key dietary considerations for individuals with type 2 diabetes:

1. **Carbohydrate Management:** Carbohydrates have the most significant effect on blood sugar levels. Managing carbohydrate intake through portion control and choosing

complex carbohydrates with a low glycemic index (GI) can help stabilize blood sugar levels and prevent spikes.

2. **Emphasis on Whole Foods:** Whole foods such as fruits, vegetables, whole grains, lean proteins, and healthy fats should form the foundation of a diabetes-friendly diet. These foods are rich in vitamins, minerals, fiber, and antioxidants, which support overall health and help regulate blood sugar levels.

3. **Limiting Added Sugars and Processed Foods:** Foods high in added sugars, refined grains, and unhealthy fats should be limited or avoided altogether. These include sugary beverages, processed snacks, fried foods, and desserts, which can contribute to insulin resistance and weight gain.

4. **Balanced Meals and Snacks:** Eating balanced meals and snacks throughout the day can help prevent blood sugar fluctuations and promote satiety. Aim for a combination of carbohydrates, proteins, and fats at each meal to maintain stable energy levels and avoid overeating.

5. **Regular Meal Timing:** Consistency in meal timing is important for individuals with type 2 diabetes to maintain stable blood sugar levels. Aim to eat meals and snacks at regular intervals throughout the day to prevent extreme fluctuations in blood glucose.

Physical Activity:

Regular physical activity is another crucial component of managing type 2 diabetes. Exercise helps improve insulin sensitivity, lower blood sugar levels, manage weight, and reduce the risk of cardiovascular complications. Here's how physical activity can benefit individuals with type 2 diabetes:

1. **Improving Insulin Sensitivity:** Exercise stimulates the uptake of glucose by muscle cells, reducing blood sugar levels and improving insulin sensitivity. Even moderate-intensity activities such as walking, swimming, or cycling can have significant benefits.

2. **Weight Management:** Physical activity plays a key role in weight management, which is particularly important for individuals with type 2 diabetes who are overweight or obese. Exercise helps burn calories, build lean muscle mass, and boost metabolism, contributing to sustainable weight loss and maintenance.

3. **Cardiovascular Health:** Regular exercise strengthens the heart, improves circulation, and lowers blood pressure and cholesterol levels, reducing the risk of cardiovascular diseases such as heart attack and stroke, which are common complications of type 2 diabetes.

4. **Stress Reduction:** Exercise is a natural stress reliever, helping to reduce cortisol levels and promote relaxation. Stress management is important for individuals with type 2 diabetes, as stress can contribute to blood sugar fluctuations and undermine overall health.

5. **Consistency and Variety:** Aim for at least 150 minutes of moderate-intensity aerobic exercise per week, spread out over several days. Incorporate a variety of activities such as brisk walking, jogging, strength training, and flexibility exercises to maximize the benefits and prevent boredom.

Weight Management:

Maintaining a healthy weight is essential for managing type 2 diabetes and reducing the risk of complications. Excess body weight, especially abdominal fat, contributes to insulin resistance and metabolic dysfunction. Here are some weight management strategies for individuals with type 2 diabetes:

1. **Calorie Control:** Achieving a calorie deficit through a combination of diet and exercise is the most effective approach to weight loss. Aim to consume fewer calories than you expend each day to promote gradual, sustainable weight loss.

2. **Portion Control:** Pay attention to portion sizes and avoid overeating, especially high-calorie foods and beverages.

Using smaller plates, measuring portions, and practicing mindful eating can help control calorie intake and prevent excess weight gain.

3. **Nutrient-Dense Foods:** Focus on nutrient-dense foods that provide essential vitamins, minerals, and fiber without excess calories. Choose whole grains, lean proteins, fruits, vegetables, and healthy fats to support overall health and satiety while managing weight.

4. **Regular Monitoring:** Keep track of your weight, food intake, physical activity, and blood sugar levels regularly to monitor progress and make necessary adjustments to your lifestyle plan. Consistent monitoring helps identify patterns, challenges, and areas for improvement.

5. **Lifestyle Modification:** Adopting healthy lifestyle habits such as regular exercise, stress management, adequate sleep, and tobacco cessation can support weight management efforts and improve overall health outcomes for individuals with type 2 diabetes.

Conclusion:

In conclusion, lifestyle factors play a critical role in managing type 2 diabetes and optimizing overall health outcomes. By making healthy dietary choices, engaging in regular physical activity, and maintaining a healthy weight, individuals with type 2 diabetes can effectively control blood sugar levels, reduce the risk of complications, and improve quality of life. It's essential to work closely with healthcare professionals, including registered dietitians, certified diabetes educators, and exercise specialists, to develop personalized lifestyle plans tailored to individual needs and preferences. With commitment, consistency, and support, adopting a healthy lifestyle can empower individuals with type 2 diabetes to take control of their health and well-being for the long term.

CHAPTER THREE

Introduction to Dr. Barbara's Simple Cure Approach

In the realm of healthcare, particularly in the context of chronic diseases like diabetes, the quest for effective treatments and management approaches is ongoing. Dr. Barbara's Simple Cure Approach offers a fresh perspective on managing diabetes by focusing on simplicity, practicality, and holistic wellness. In this introduction, we'll explore the foundational principles of Dr. Barbara's approach and its potential benefits for individuals with diabetes.

Understanding the Need for Simplicity:

Managing diabetes can often feel overwhelming, with a multitude of medications, dietary guidelines, and lifestyle recommendations to navigate. Dr. Barbara's Simple Cure Approach recognizes the complexity of diabetes management and emphasizes the importance of simplifying the process for patients. By distilling complex medical concepts into straightforward guidelines and actionable steps, Dr. Barbara aims to empower individuals with diabetes to take control of their health with confidence and ease.

Holistic Wellness as a Core Principle:

Dr. Barbara's approach to diabetes management extends beyond conventional medical interventions to embrace the concept of holistic wellness. Recognizing the interconnectedness of physical, emotional, and spiritual well-being, Dr. Barbara advocates for a comprehensive approach that addresses all aspects of health. This holistic perspective acknowledges the impact of lifestyle factors, stress, mental health, and social support on diabetes management outcomes.

Key Components of Dr. Barbara's Simple Cure Approach:

1. **Personalized Care Plans:** Dr. Barbara believes in the importance of personalized care plans tailored to each individual's unique needs, preferences, and circumstances. Rather than adopting a one-size-fits-all approach, she emphasizes the importance of collaboration between patients and healthcare providers to develop customized strategies for managing diabetes effectively.

2. **Emphasis on Lifestyle Modification:** Central to Dr. Barbara's Simple Cure Approach is the recognition of the profound influence of lifestyle factors on diabetes management outcomes. She advocates for simple yet impactful lifestyle modifications, including dietary changes, regular physical activity, stress management techniques, and adequate sleep. These lifestyle interventions are aimed at improving blood sugar control, promoting weight management, and reducing the risk of complications.

3. **Focus on Education and Empowerment:** Education is a cornerstone of Dr. Barbara's approach, empowering individuals with diabetes with the knowledge and skills they need to make informed decisions about their health. Through clear and accessible educational materials, Dr. Barbara demystifies medical jargon and equips patients with practical tools for self-care, monitoring, and problem-solving.

4. **Integration of Complementary Therapies:** Dr. Barbara recognizes the potential benefits of complementary therapies in supporting conventional diabetes management strategies. While emphasizing the importance of evidence-based practices, she encourages exploration of complementary modalities such as acupuncture, yoga, meditation, and herbal remedies under the guidance of qualified practitioners.

5. **Promotion of Positive Mindset and Self-Compassion:** Dr. Barbara emphasizes the importance of cultivating a positive mindset and practicing self-compassion in the journey of managing diabetes. She acknowledges the emotional challenges and frustrations that individuals with diabetes may face and encourages a non-judgmental and supportive approach to self-care.

Conclusion:

In conclusion, Dr. Barbara's Simple Cure Approach offers a refreshing perspective on managing diabetes that prioritizes simplicity, holistic wellness, and patient empowerment. By focusing on personalized care plans, lifestyle modification, education, and integration of complementary therapies, Dr. Barbara aims to empower individuals with diabetes to achieve optimal health and well-being. Through a combination of practical guidance, emotional support, and empowerment, Dr. Barbara's approach seeks to transform the experience of living with diabetes from one of complexity and uncertainty to one of simplicity and confidence.

CHAPTER FOUR

Key Principles of Dr. Barbara's Diabetes Treatment Protocol

Dr. Barbara's Diabetes Treatment Protocol is grounded in a holistic approach to managing diabetes that emphasizes simplicity, empowerment, and comprehensive wellness. Through a combination of evidence-based practices, personalized care plans, and patient education, Dr. Barbara's protocol aims to optimize blood sugar control, prevent complications, and improve overall quality of life for individuals living with diabetes. Below are the key principles that underpin Dr. Barbara's approach:

1. Personalized Care Plans: Dr. Barbara recognizes that each individual with diabetes is unique, with distinct health needs, preferences, and circumstances. Therefore, her treatment protocol emphasizes the importance of developing personalized care plans tailored to the specific needs of each patient. These care plans take into account factors such as age, gender, medical history, lifestyle, cultural background, and treatment goals. By customizing care plans, Dr. Barbara aims to optimize treatment outcomes and empower patients to actively participate in their own care.

2. Holistic Wellness: A core principle of Dr. Barbara's treatment protocol is the recognition of the interconnectedness of physical, emotional, and spiritual well-being. Rather than focusing solely on managing blood sugar levels, her approach encompasses a holistic view of health that addresses the whole person. This includes promoting healthy lifestyle habits, managing stress, fostering positive relationships, and nurturing emotional resilience. By prioritizing holistic wellness, Dr. Barbara aims to improve overall health outcomes and enhance quality of life for individuals with diabetes.

3. Lifestyle Modification: Dr. Barbara's treatment protocol places a strong emphasis on lifestyle modification as a cornerstone of diabetes management. This includes making healthy dietary choices, engaging in regular physical activity, maintaining a healthy weight, managing stress effectively, and getting adequate sleep. Lifestyle modification is essential for optimizing blood sugar control, reducing the risk of complications, and improving long-term health outcomes. Dr. Barbara provides practical guidance and support to help patients implement sustainable lifestyle changes that promote health and well-being.

4. Patient Education and Empowerment: Education is a central component of Dr. Barbara's treatment protocol, empowering patients with the knowledge and skills they need to manage their diabetes effectively. Through clear and accessible educational materials, individualized counseling sessions, and ongoing support, Dr. Barbara helps patients understand their condition, treatment options, and self-care strategies. By empowering patients to take an active role in their own care, Dr. Barbara fosters a sense of ownership, confidence, and self-efficacy.

5. Regular Monitoring and Follow-Up: Dr. Barbara emphasizes the importance of regular monitoring and follow-up to track progress, identify any potential issues, and make necessary adjustments to treatment plans. This includes monitoring blood sugar levels, tracking dietary and lifestyle habits, assessing medication adherence, and evaluating overall health status. Regular check-ins with healthcare providers allow for ongoing support, guidance, and optimization of treatment strategies based on individual needs and responses.

6. Integration of Complementary Therapies: Dr. Barbara's treatment protocol recognizes the potential benefits of integrating complementary therapies into diabetes management strategies. While emphasizing the importance of evidence-based practices, she acknowledges that complementary modalities such as acupuncture, yoga, meditation, and herbal remedies may offer additional support in managing diabetes-related symptoms, improving overall well-being, and enhancing quality of life. Dr. Barbara encourages patients to explore these complementary therapies under the guidance of qualified practitioners and in conjunction with conventional medical treatments.

In summary, Dr. Barbara's Diabetes Treatment Protocol embodies key principles of personalized care, holistic wellness, lifestyle modification, patient education, regular monitoring, and integration of complementary therapies. By adopting a comprehensive approach that addresses the unique needs of each individual with diabetes, Dr. Barbara aims to empower patients to achieve optimal health outcomes and live fulfilling lives despite their diagnosis.

CHAPTER FIVE

Herbal Remedies for Blood Sugar Control and Insulin Sensitivity

Herbal remedies have been used for centuries in traditional medicine systems around the world to manage various health conditions, including diabetes. While scientific research on the effectiveness of herbal remedies for blood sugar control and insulin sensitivity is ongoing, some herbs have shown promising results in clinical studies. It's essential to approach herbal remedies with caution and consult with a healthcare professional before incorporating them into your diabetes management plan, especially if you're already taking medications or have other health conditions. Here are some herbal remedies that have been studied for their potential benefits in blood sugar control and insulin sensitivity:

1. Cinnamon (Cinnamomum verum, Cinnamomum cassia): Cinnamon is a popular spice that has been investigated for its potential hypoglycemic effects. Some studies suggest that cinnamon may help improve insulin sensitivity and lower blood sugar levels by enhancing glucose uptake in cells. However, results from clinical trials have been mixed, and more research is needed to determine the optimal dose and long-term effects of cinnamon supplementation on diabetes management.

2. Gymnema Sylvestre: Gymnemasylvestre, also known as gurmar, is an herb native to India and has a long history of use in Ayurvedic medicine for its anti-diabetic properties. Research suggests that gymnemasylvestre may help lower blood sugar levels by blocking sugar absorption in the intestines and increasing insulin production in the pancreas. Some studies have also reported improvements in insulin sensitivity and glycemic control with gymnemasylvestre supplementation.

3. Bitter Melon (Momordica charantia): Bitter melon is a tropical fruit that is commonly used in traditional medicine for its anti-diabetic properties. It contains compounds that may help improve blood sugar control and increase insulin sensitivity. Research suggests that bitter melon supplementation may reduce fasting blood sugar levels and improve glucose tolerance in individuals with type 2 diabetes. However, more high-quality studies are needed to confirm its effectiveness and safety.

4. Fenugreek (Trigonella foenum-graecum): Fenugreek seeds are rich in soluble fiber and other bioactive compounds that may help regulate blood sugar levels and improve insulin sensitivity. Studies have shown that fenugreek supplementation may lead to reductions in fasting blood sugar levels, postprandial glucose levels, and HbA1c levels in individuals with type 2 diabetes. Fenugreek may also have beneficial effects on lipid profiles and cardiovascular health.

5. Ginseng (Panax ginseng, Panax quinquefolius): Ginseng is an herb that has been used in traditional Chinese medicine for its adaptogenic and anti-diabetic properties. Research suggests that ginseng may help improve insulin sensitivity, enhance glucose metabolism, and reduce oxidative stress in individuals with type 2 diabetes. However, the evidence is mixed, and more studies are needed to clarify the role of ginseng in diabetes management.

6. Berberine: Berberine is a bioactive compound found in several plants, including goldenseal, Oregon grape, and barberry. It has been studied extensively for its potential therapeutic effects on blood sugar control and insulin sensitivity. Research suggests that berberine may help lower blood sugar levels, improve insulin sensitivity, and reduce HbA1c levels in individuals with type 2 diabetes. It may also have beneficial effects on lipid metabolism and cardiovascular health.

7. Aloe Vera: Aloe vera is a succulent plant that has been used in traditional medicine for its various health benefits, including its potential anti-diabetic effects. Studies suggest that aloe vera supplementation may help lower fasting blood sugar levels and HbA1c levels in individuals with type 2 diabetes. It may also have antioxidant and anti-inflammatory properties that contribute to its therapeutic effects.

While these herbal remedies show promise in improving blood sugar control and insulin sensitivity, it's important to remember that they are not meant to replace conventional diabetes medications or lifestyle interventions. Additionally, herbal remedies can interact with medications and may not be safe for everyone, especially pregnant or breastfeeding women, individuals with certain medical conditions, or those taking specific medications. Therefore, it's crucial to consult with a healthcare professional before starting any herbal supplementation regimen to ensure safety and efficacy.

CHAPTER SIX

Nutritional Strategies for Managing Type 2 Diabetes

Nutritional strategies play a crucial role in managing type 2 diabetes, as diet has a direct impact on blood sugar levels, insulin sensitivity, and overall health outcomes. By adopting a balanced and individualized approach to nutrition, individuals with type 2 diabetes can effectively manage their condition, prevent complications, and improve quality of life. Here are some key nutritional strategies for managing type 2 diabetes:

1. Emphasize Whole Foods: Focus on consuming a variety of whole, minimally processed foods that are rich in nutrients and fiber. These include fruits, vegetables, whole grains, legumes, lean proteins, and healthy fats. Whole foods provide essential vitamins, minerals, antioxidants, and fiber, which support overall health and help regulate blood sugar levels.

2. Monitor Carbohydrate Intake: Carbohydrates have the most significant impact on blood sugar levels, so it's important to monitor carbohydrate intake and choose carbohydrates wisely. Focus on consuming complex carbohydrates with a low glycemic index (GI), such as whole grains, legumes, fruits, and vegetables, which are digested more slowly and have less of an impact on blood sugar levels. Limit or avoid refined carbohydrates and sugary foods and beverages, which can cause spikes in blood sugar levels.

3. Practice Portion Control: Be mindful of portion sizes to prevent overeating and manage blood sugar levels. Use measuring cups, food scales, or visual cues to portion out foods, especially carbohydrate-rich foods. Aim for balanced meals that include a combination of carbohydrates, proteins, and fats to help stabilize blood sugar levels and promote satiety.

4. Choose Healthy Fats: Include sources of healthy fats in your diet, such as avocados, nuts, seeds, olive oil, and fatty fish. Healthy fats help improve insulin sensitivity, regulate blood sugar levels, and support heart health. Limit saturated and trans fats found in fried foods, processed snacks, and fatty meats, as they can increase the risk of cardiovascular disease.

5. Prioritize Protein: Include lean sources of protein in your meals and snacks to help stabilize blood sugar levels and promote satiety. Good sources of protein include poultry, fish, tofu, tempeh, legumes, and low-fat dairy products. Spread protein intake throughout the day to support muscle maintenance and repair.

6. Focus on Timing and Balance: Space out meals and snacks evenly throughout the day to prevent extreme fluctuations in blood sugar levels. Aim for three balanced meals and 1-2 snacks per day, with carbohydrates distributed evenly across meals.

Include a source of protein and healthy fat with each meal to help slow the digestion and absorption of carbohydrates.

7. Stay Hydrated: Drink plenty of water throughout the day to stay hydrated and support overall health. Limit sugary beverages such as soda, fruit juice, and sweetened drinks, as they can contribute to blood sugar spikes and provide empty calories. Opt for water, herbal tea, or sparkling water with lemon or lime for a refreshing and hydrating alternative.

8. Monitor Blood Sugar Levels: Regularly monitor your blood sugar levels using a glucometer or continuous glucose monitor (CGM) to track how different foods and lifestyle choices affect your blood sugar levels. Keep a record of your blood sugar readings, meals, physical activity, medications, and other relevant factors to identify patterns and make informed adjustments to your diabetes management plan.

9. Seek Professional Guidance: Consult with a registered dietitian or certified diabetes educator to develop a personalized nutrition plan tailored to your individual needs, preferences, and health goals. A healthcare professional can provide evidence-based guidance, practical tips, and ongoing support to help you make healthy dietary choices and effectively manage your type 2 diabetes.

By implementing these nutritional strategies and making healthy lifestyle choices, individuals with type 2 diabetes can improve blood sugar control, reduce the risk of complications, and enhance overall health and well-being. It's important to approach nutrition as part of a comprehensive diabetes management plan that also includes regular physical activity, medication management, stress reduction, and regular monitoring of blood sugar levels. With dedication, consistency, and support, managing type 2 diabetes through nutrition can lead to better health outcomes and a higher quality of life.

CHAPTER SEVEN

Incorporating Physical Activity into Your Diabetes Management Plan

Incorporating physical activity into your diabetes management plan is essential for maintaining good health, managing blood sugar levels, and reducing the risk of complications associated with type 2 diabetes. Regular exercise offers numerous benefits, including improved insulin sensitivity, weight management, cardiovascular health, stress reduction, and enhanced overall well-being. Here are some key considerations and practical tips for incorporating physical activity into your diabetes management plan:

1. Consult with Your Healthcare Team: Before starting any exercise program, it's important to consult with your healthcare team, including your doctor and a certified diabetes educator. They can assess your current health status, provide personalized recommendations, and help you develop a safe and effective exercise plan based on your individual needs, fitness level, and medical history.

2. Set Realistic Goals: Set realistic and achievable goals for your physical activity regimen based on your current fitness level, health status, and personal preferences. Start with small, manageable goals and gradually increase the intensity, duration, and frequency of your workouts as you progress. Celebrate your achievements along the way to stay motivated and committed to your exercise routine.

3. Choose Activities You Enjoy: Select physical activities that you enjoy and look forward to doing on a regular basis. Whether it's walking, cycling, swimming, dancing, gardening, or playing a sport, find activities that you find fun and engaging. This will help you stay motivated, sustain your interest in exercise, and make it easier to stick to your diabetes management plan in the long term.

4. Make Exercise a Priority: Make exercise a priority in your daily routine by scheduling it into your calendar and treating it like any other important appointment. Aim for at least 150 minutes of moderate-intensity aerobic exercise per week, spread out over several days. You can also incorporate strength training exercises at least two days a week to build muscle mass, improve metabolism, and enhance overall fitness.

5. Start Slow and Gradually Increase Intensity: If you're new to exercise or have been inactive for a while, start slow and gradually increase the intensity and duration of your workouts over time. Begin with low-impact activities and gradually progress to higher-intensity exercises as your fitness level improves. Listen to your body and adjust your exercise intensity based on how you feel to avoid overexertion or injury.

6. Monitor Your Blood Sugar Levels: Monitor your blood sugar levels before, during, and after exercise to understand how physical activity affects your glucose levels. Keep track of any changes in blood sugar levels and adjust your diabetes management plan accordingly, such as adjusting your carbohydrate intake or medication doses as needed. Be prepared to treat and prevent hypoglycemia (low blood sugar) during and after exercise by carrying glucose tablets or snacks with you.

7. Stay Hydrated and Fuel Your Body: Stay hydrated before, during, and after exercise by drinking plenty of water or other hydrating fluids. It's also important to fuel your body with nutritious foods before and after exercise to support energy levels, muscle recovery, and overall performance. Eat a balanced meal or snack that includes carbohydrates, protein, and healthy fats to provide sustained energy and promote muscle repair and growth.

8. Listen to Your Body and Rest When Needed: Pay attention to how your body feels during and after exercise and listen to any warning signs or signals of fatigue, pain, or discomfort. Allow yourself time to rest and recover between workouts to prevent overtraining and reduce the risk of injury. Incorporate rest days into your exercise routine and prioritize adequate sleep to support overall health and well-being.

9. Stay Consistent and Be Patient: Consistency is key when it comes to reaping the benefits of physical activity for diabetes management. Stay committed to your exercise routine, even on days when you may not feel motivated or energized. Be patient with yourself and recognize that progress takes time. Focus on making small, sustainable changes and celebrate your accomplishments along the way.

By incorporating physical activity into your diabetes management plan, you can improve blood sugar control, enhance overall health and well-being, and reduce the risk of complications associated with type 2 diabetes. Remember to consult with your healthcare team before starting any exercise program and tailor your physical activity regimen to your individual needs, preferences, and goals. With dedication, consistency, and support, regular exercise can become a rewarding and enjoyable part of your diabetes management plan.

CHAPTER EIGHT

Mind-Body Techniques for Stress Reduction and Blood Sugar Regulation

Mind-body techniques offer effective strategies for reducing stress and promoting blood sugar regulation in individuals with type 2 diabetes. Chronic stress can negatively impact blood sugar levels by triggering the release of stress hormones such as cortisol and adrenaline, which can lead to insulin resistance and glucose dysregulation. By incorporating mind-body techniques into your diabetes management plan, you can effectively manage stress, improve insulin sensitivity, and enhance overall well-being. Here are some mind-body techniques to consider:

1. Meditation: Meditation is a powerful practice that can help calm the mind, reduce stress, and promote relaxation. Mindfulness meditation, in particular, involves focusing your attention on the present moment without judgment, which can help alleviate anxiety and promote a sense of inner peace. Regular meditation practice has been shown to improve blood sugar control, reduce HbA1c levels, and enhance overall psychological well-being in individuals with type 2 diabetes.

2. Deep Breathing Exercises: Deep breathing exercises, such as diaphragmatic breathing or belly breathing, can help activate the body's relaxation response and reduce stress levels. By focusing on slow, deep breaths and engaging the diaphragm, you can lower cortisol levels, decrease heart rate, and promote feelings of calmness and relaxation. Incorporate deep breathing exercises into your daily routine, especially during times of stress or before meals, to support blood sugar regulation and overall health.

3. Progressive Muscle Relaxation (PMR): Progressive muscle relaxation is a technique that involves tensing and relaxing different muscle groups in the body to release tension and promote relaxation. By systematically tensing and releasing muscle groups from head to toe, you can reduce physical and mental stress, alleviate muscle tension, and improve overall well-being. Practice PMR regularly to reduce stress levels and support blood sugar regulation in individuals with type 2 diabetes.

4. Yoga: Yoga is a mind-body practice that combines physical postures, breath control, and meditation to promote relaxation, flexibility, and inner peace. Regular yoga practice has been shown to reduce stress, improve insulin sensitivity, and enhance overall health outcomes in individuals with type 2 diabetes. Choose gentle or restorative yoga classes that focus on relaxation and mindfulness to support stress reduction and blood sugar regulation.

5. Tai Chi: Tai Chi is a gentle form of martial arts that emphasizes slow, flowing movements and deep breathing to promote relaxation, balance, and harmony in the body and mind. Regular practice of Tai Chi has been shown to reduce stress, improve insulin sensitivity, and enhance cardiovascular health in individuals with type 2 diabetes. Incorporate Tai Chi into your exercise routine as a low-impact activity that supports stress reduction and overall well-being.

6. Guided Imagery: Guided imagery involves using visualization techniques to create mental images that promote relaxation and reduce stress. By imagining peaceful scenes or positive outcomes, you can shift your focus away from stressors and promote feelings of calmness and well-being. Practice guided imagery regularly, either on your own or with the guidance of a trained therapist or audio recording, to support stress reduction and blood sugar regulation.

7. Biofeedback: Biofeedback is a technique that allows individuals to monitor and control their physiological responses, such as heart rate, blood pressure, and muscle tension, through real-time feedback. By learning to regulate these responses, you can reduce stress levels, promote relaxation, and improve overall health outcomes. Work with a trained therapist or use biofeedback devices to learn how to control your body's stress response and support blood sugar regulation.

Incorporating mind-body techniques into your diabetes management plan can help reduce stress, promote relaxation, and improve blood sugar regulation in individuals with type 2 diabetes. Experiment with different techniques to find what works best for you, and integrate them into your daily routine to support overall well-being and diabetes management. Remember to consult with your healthcare team before starting any new stress management techniques, especially if you have any underlying health conditions or concerns.

CHAPTER NINE

Monitoring Progress and Adjusting Your Treatment Plan

Monitoring progress and adjusting your treatment plan are essential components of managing type 2 diabetes effectively. Regular monitoring allows you to track changes in your blood sugar levels, assess the effectiveness of your current treatment regimen, and make necessary adjustments to optimize your diabetes management plan. Here are some key steps for monitoring progress and adjusting your treatment plan:

1. Blood Sugar Monitoring: Regular blood sugar monitoring is crucial for individuals with type 2 diabetes to track their glucose levels and identify patterns over time. Monitor your blood sugar levels according to your healthcare provider's recommendations, which may include fasting blood glucose, postprandial (after-meal) glucose, and periodic HbA1c tests. Keep a log of your blood sugar readings, along with details such as meals, physical activity, medication doses, and any symptoms you experience.

2. Lifestyle Assessment: Evaluate your current lifestyle habits, including diet, physical activity, stress management, sleep quality, and medication adherence. Assess how these factors are impacting your blood sugar levels, overall health, and well-being. Identify areas where you can make improvements and set specific goals for diet, exercise, stress reduction, and medication management based on your individual needs and preferences.

3. Consult with Your Healthcare Team: Schedule regular check-ups with your healthcare team, including your doctor, registered dietitian, diabetes educator, and other specialists as needed. Review your blood sugar monitoring data, lifestyle habits, medication regimen, and any concerns or challenges you may be facing. Discuss your treatment goals, progress, and preferences with your healthcare team to develop a collaborative approach to managing your type 2 diabetes.

4. Adjust Medications as Needed: If your blood sugar levels are consistently above or below your target range despite lifestyle modifications, your healthcare provider may recommend adjusting your medication regimen. This may involve changing the type, dose, or timing of your medications to better control your blood sugar levels and minimize the risk of complications. Follow your healthcare provider's recommendations and monitor your response to medication adjustments closely.

5. Implement Lifestyle Modifications: Make gradual changes to your diet, physical activity, stress management, and sleep habits based on your treatment goals and healthcare provider's recommendations. Focus on incorporating sustainable lifestyle modifications that promote blood sugar control, weight management, cardiovascular health, and overall well-being.

Monitor your progress and adjust your lifestyle plan as needed to achieve optimal results.

6. Monitor for Symptoms and Complications: Be vigilant for any symptoms or signs of complications associated with type 2 diabetes, such as increased thirst, frequent urination, fatigue, blurred vision, slow wound healing, or numbness or tingling in the hands and feet. Report any changes or concerns to your healthcare provider promptly to prevent or manage potential complications and ensure timely intervention.

7. Stay Educated and Empowered: Educate yourself about type 2 diabetes, its management, and the importance of self-care and monitoring. Stay informed about new research, treatment options, and lifestyle strategies for managing diabetes effectively. Take an active role in your diabetes management plan, ask questions, seek support from your healthcare team and peers, and advocate for your health needs and preferences.

8. Celebrate Achievements and Stay Positive: Celebrate your achievements, no matter how small, and acknowledge the progress you've made towards your treatment goals. Stay positive and resilient in the face of challenges, setbacks, and fluctuations in blood sugar levels. Remember that managing type 2 diabetes is a journey, and your healthcare team is there to support you every step of the way.

By monitoring progress, adjusting your treatment plan as needed, and staying proactive and engaged in your diabetes management, you can effectively control your blood sugar levels, reduce the risk of complications, and improve your overall health and well-being. Regular communication with your healthcare team, adherence to treatment recommendations, and commitment to a healthy lifestyle are key factors in achieving optimal outcomes in managing type 2 diabetes.

CHAPTER TEN

Long-Term Maintenance: Sustaining Healthy Habits and Preventing Complications

Long-term maintenance is crucial for individuals with type 2 diabetes to sustain healthy habits, prevent complications, and achieve optimal health outcomes over time. Managing type 2 diabetes is a lifelong journey that requires ongoing commitment, vigilance, and support. Here are some key strategies for sustaining healthy habits and preventing complications in the long term:

1. Commit to Healthy Lifestyle Habits: Maintain a commitment to healthy lifestyle habits, including a balanced diet, regular physical activity, stress management, adequate sleep, and avoiding smoking and excessive alcohol consumption. These habits play a central role in managing blood sugar levels, promoting overall health, and reducing the risk of complications associated with type 2 diabetes.

2. Follow a Balanced Diet: Continue to follow a balanced and nutritious diet that emphasizes whole foods, such as fruits, vegetables, whole grains, lean proteins, and healthy fats. Monitor portion sizes, carbohydrate intake, and meal timing to help regulate blood sugar levels and support weight management. Consider consulting with a registered dietitian or certified diabetes educator for personalized nutrition guidance and meal planning strategies.

3. Stay Active: Maintain regular physical activity as part of your daily routine to support blood sugar control, cardiovascular health, weight management, and overall well-being. Aim for at least 150 minutes of moderate-intensity aerobic exercise per week, along with strength training exercises at least two days a week. Find activities you enjoy and make physical activity a priority in your schedule.

4. Monitor Blood Sugar Levels: Continue to monitor your blood sugar levels regularly as recommended by your healthcare provider, using glucometers, continuous glucose monitors (CGMs), or other monitoring devices. Keep track of your blood sugar readings, patterns, and trends over time to identify any changes or fluctuations. Use this information to make informed decisions about your diabetes management plan and adjust your treatment regimen as needed.

5. Adhere to Medication and Treatment Recommendations: Follow your healthcare provider's recommendations for medication adherence, including taking prescribed medications as directed, monitoring for side effects or interactions, and attending regular check-ups and follow-up appointments. Communicate openly with your healthcare team about any concerns or challenges you may encounter, and work together to optimize your treatment plan for long-term success.

6. Manage Stress Effectively: Practice stress management techniques, such as mindfulness meditation, deep breathing exercises, yoga, tai chi, progressive muscle relaxation, or guided imagery, to reduce stress levels and promote relaxation. Find healthy ways to cope with stressors in your life and prioritize self-care activities that promote mental and emotional well-being.

7. Educate Yourself and Stay Informed: Stay educated about type 2 diabetes, its management, and the latest research and developments in diabetes care. Take advantage of educational resources, support groups, online forums, and community programs to learn more about diabetes management, share experiences, and connect with others who understand what you're going through.

8. Monitor for Signs of Complications: Be vigilant for any signs or symptoms of complications associated with type 2 diabetes, such as neuropathy, retinopathy, nephropathy, cardiovascular disease, or foot problems. Report any changes or concerns to your healthcare provider promptly for early detection, intervention, and management of complications.

9. Cultivate a Supportive Network: Surround yourself with a supportive network of family members, friends, healthcare providers, and peers who understand and support your journey with type 2 diabetes. Seek encouragement, advice, and guidance from others who can offer empathy, understanding, and practical support when needed.

10. Stay Positive and Resilient: Maintain a positive outlook and cultivate resilience in the face of challenges, setbacks, or fluctuations in blood sugar levels. Focus on the progress you've made, celebrate your achievements, and learn from any obstacles or setbacks along the way. Stay motivated and committed to your long-term health and well-being, knowing that you have the knowledge, skills, and support to manage type 2 diabetes effectively.

By adopting these strategies for long-term maintenance, individuals with type 2 diabetes can sustain healthy habits, prevent complications, and achieve optimal health outcomes over time. Remember that managing type 2 diabetes is a journey, and each day presents an opportunity to make positive choices that support your overall health and well-being. Stay proactive, informed, and empowered in managing your diabetes, and don't hesitate to reach out to your healthcare team for support and guidance along the way.

SOME HERBAL REMEDIES FOR TYPE 2 DIABETES

1. Bitter Melon (Momordica charantia)

Definition: Bitter melon is a tropical vine with edible fruit that has a distinct bitter taste and medicinal properties known to help manage blood sugar levels.

- **Ingredients:** Fresh bitter melon fruit or bitter melon powder.

- **How to Prepare:** For fresh fruit, wash, cut, and remove seeds. Blend into juice or cook in dishes. For powder, mix with water.

- **How to Use:** Drink bitter melon juice or incorporate the vegetable into meals.

- **Dosage:** 50-100 ml of juice daily or as recommended by a healthcare provider.

- **Side Effects:** Nausea, vomiting, diarrhea, and abdominal pain.

- **Precautions:** Avoid if pregnant or breastfeeding, as it may induce labor or affect milk production.

2. Fenugreek (Trigonella foenum-graecum)

Definition: Fenugreek is a herb with seeds known for their ability to help regulate blood sugar.

- **Ingredients:** Fenugreek seeds or powder.

- **How to Prepare:** Soak seeds overnight or grind into powder.

- **How to Use:** Consume soaked seeds or mix powder with water or food.

- **Dosage:** 5-10 grams daily.

- **Side Effects:** Gastrointestinal issues like gas, bloating, and diarrhea.

- **Precautions:** Consult a doctor if pregnant or taking other medications, as it may interfere with absorption.

3. Ginseng (Panax ginseng)

Definition: Ginseng is a root traditionally used in Chinese medicine to help stabilize blood sugar.

- **Ingredients:** Ginseng root or extract.

- **How to Prepare:** Brew tea from the root or take as a capsule/extract.

- **How to Use:** Drink ginseng tea or take supplements.

- **Dosage:** 200-400 mg of extract daily.

- **Side Effects:** Insomnia, headaches, dizziness, and digestive issues.

- **Precautions:** Avoid use with other stimulants or if you have heart problems.

4. Cinnamon (Cinnamomum verum)

Definition: Cinnamon is a spice derived from the bark of the cinnamon tree, known for its blood sugar-lowering effects.

- **Ingredients:** Cinnamon sticks, powder, or extract.

- **How to Prepare:** Add to food, beverages, or take as a supplement.

- **How to Use:** Sprinkle on food or brew as tea.

- **Dosage:** 1-6 grams daily.

- **Side Effects:** Liver issues in high doses, allergic reactions.

- **Precautions:** Consult a doctor if you have liver disease or are pregnant.

5. Aloe Vera (Aloe barbadensis)

Definition: Aloe vera is a succulent plant whose gel is used for various medicinal purposes, including diabetes management.

- **Ingredients:** Fresh aloe vera leaves or commercial aloe vera gel.

- **How to Prepare:** Extract gel from fresh leaves.

- **How to Use:** Consume gel directly or mix with water/juice.

- **Dosage:** 1-2 tablespoons daily.

- **Side Effects:** Gastrointestinal discomfort, electrolyte imbalance.

- **Precautions:** Avoid long-term use due to potential kidney issues.

6. Berberine

Definition: Berberine is a compound found in several plants, including goldenseal and barberry, known for its glucose-lowering properties.

- **Ingredients:** Berberine extract.

- **How to Prepare:** Available in capsule or powder form.

- **How to Use:** Take as a supplement.

- **Dosage:** 500 mg, 2-3 times daily.

- **Side Effects:** Digestive issues, low blood pressure.

- **Precautions:** May interact with medications; consult a doctor.

7. Turmeric (Curcuma longa)

Definition: Turmeric is a spice with anti-inflammatory properties that may help manage diabetes.

- **Ingredients:** Turmeric powder or fresh turmeric root.

- **How to Prepare:** Add to food, beverages, or take as a supplement.

- **How to Use:** Incorporate into meals or drink turmeric tea.

- **Dosage:** 500-2000 mg daily.

- **Side Effects:** Gastrointestinal issues, gallbladder problems.

- **Precautions:** Avoid if you have gallbladder disease.

8. Gymnema Sylvestre

Definition: Gymnema is a herb used in traditional medicine to lower blood sugar.

- **Ingredients:** Gymnema leaves or extract.

- **How to Prepare:** Brew leaves as tea or take as a supplement.

- **How to Use:** Drink tea or take capsules.

- **Dosage:** 200-400 mg of extract daily.

- **Side Effects:** Hypoglycemia, digestive issues.

- **Precautions:** Monitor blood sugar levels closely.

9. Holy Basil (Ocimum sanctum)

Definition: Holy basil is an herb with anti-diabetic properties, used in Ayurvedic medicine.

- **Ingredients:** Fresh holy basil leaves or dried leaves.

- **How to Prepare:** Brew leaves as tea or consume fresh.

- **How to Use:** Drink tea or chew fresh leaves.

- **Dosage:** 2-5 leaves daily or one cup of tea.

- **Side Effects:** Mild nausea or discomfort.

- **Precautions:** Safe for most, but consult a doctor if pregnant or breastfeeding.

10. Neem (Azadirachta indica)

Definition: Neem is a tree whose leaves and bark are used in traditional medicine to manage diabetes.

- **Ingredients:** Neem leaves or extract.

- **How to Prepare:** Brew leaves as tea or take as a supplement.

- **How to Use:** Drink neem tea or take capsules.

- **Dosage:** 5 grams of leaves daily or as recommended.

- **Side Effects:** Liver damage in high doses, stomach irritation.

- **Precautions:** Avoid during pregnancy and breastfeeding.

11. Bilberry (Vaccinium myrtillus)

Definition: Bilberry is a berry similar to blueberry, used to manage blood sugar levels.

- **Ingredients:** Fresh bilberries, dried berries, or extract.
- **How to Prepare:** Consume fresh berries, brew dried berries as tea, or take extract.
- **How to Use:** Eat berries or drink tea.
- **Dosage:** 20-60 grams of fresh berries or 160 mg of extract daily.
- **Side Effects:** Mild digestive issues.
- **Precautions:** Safe in moderate amounts; consult a doctor if taking blood-thinning medications.

12. Ginger (Zingiber officinale)

Definition: Ginger is a root with anti-inflammatory and blood sugar-lowering properties.

- **Ingredients:** Fresh ginger root or ginger powder.
- **How to Prepare:** Brew as tea or add to food.
- **How to Use:** Drink ginger tea or incorporate into meals.
- **Dosage:** 2-4 grams daily.
- **Side Effects:** Heartburn, diarrhea.

- **Precautions:** May interact with blood thinners; consult a doctor.

13. Milk Thistle (Silybum marianum)

Definition: Milk thistle is a flowering herb known for its liver-protective and blood sugar-regulating effects.

- **Ingredients:** Milk thistle seeds or extract.

- **How to Prepare:** Brew seeds as tea or take extract.

- **How to Use:** Drink milk thistle tea or take capsules.

- **Dosage:** 200-300 mg of extract daily.

- **Side Effects:** Gastrointestinal issues, allergic reactions.

- **Precautions:** Consult a doctor if pregnant or breastfeeding.

14. Green Tea (Camellia sinensis)

Definition: Green tea is made from unoxidized tea leaves and has antioxidants that help manage blood sugar.

- **Ingredients:** Green tea leaves or bags.

- **How to Prepare:** Brew leaves or bags in hot water.

- **How to Use:** Drink green tea.

- **Dosage:** 3-4 cups daily.

- **Side Effects:** Caffeine-related issues like insomnia or jitteriness.

- **Precautions:** Limit if sensitive to caffeine or pregnant.

15. Dandelion (Taraxacum officinale)

Definition: Dandelion is a plant whose root and leaves are used for their medicinal properties, including blood sugar regulation.

- **Ingredients:** Dandelion root or leaves.

- **How to Prepare:** Brew root or leaves as tea.

- **How to Use:** Drink dandelion tea.

- **Dosage:** 1-2 cups of tea daily.

- **Side Effects:** Gastrointestinal issues, allergic reactions.

- **Precautions:** Avoid if allergic to dandelions or related plants.

General Precautions:

- Always consult with a healthcare provider before starting any herbal remedy, especially if you are on medication or have other health conditions.

- Monitor blood sugar levels regularly to avoid hypoglycemia.

- Pregnant or breastfeeding women should be particularly cautious and seek medical advice before using herbal remedies.

BONUS

SOME ESSENTIAL HOLISTIC REMEDIES TO KNOW

Cell Food:

Definition: Cell Food is a dietary supplement marketed as a highly oxygenating and alkalizing formula. It's claimed to support overall health and vitality by providing essential nutrients and oxygen to the cells.

Ingredients: The exact ingredients of Cell Food can vary depending on the brand, but it typically contains a proprietary blend of minerals, enzymes, electrolytes, and trace elements. Some common ingredients may include purified water, dissolved oxygen, seawater extract, and plant-based enzymes.

How to Prepare: Cell Food is usually available in liquid form and is typically taken orally. It can be consumed directly or diluted in water or juice before consumption.

Dosage: The dosage of Cell Food can vary depending on the specific product and individual needs. It's important to follow the recommended dosage on the product label or consult with a healthcare professional for personalized guidance.

How to Use: Cell Food is typically taken orally, either directly or mixed into water or juice. It's important to shake the bottle well before use and to store it according to the manufacturer's instructions.

Side Effects: Cell Food is generally considered safe for most people when used as directed. However, some individuals may experience mild digestive upset or allergic reactions to certain ingredients. It's essential to consult with a healthcare provider before starting any new supplement regimen, especially if you have underlying health conditions or are taking medications.

Chaparral:

Definition: Chaparral, scientifically known as Larrea tridentata, is a shrub native to the southwestern United States and northern Mexico. It has been used for centuries by Native American tribes for its medicinal properties and is commonly used in herbal medicine today.

Ingredients: Chaparral contains several bioactive compounds, including nordihydroguaiaretic acid (NDGA), flavonoids, lignans, and volatile oils. NDGA is believed to be the primary active compound responsible for many of chaparral's therapeutic effects.

How to Prepare: Chaparral can be prepared and consumed in various forms, including teas, tinctures, capsules, and topical preparations. To make tea, dried chaparral leaves are steeped in hot water for several minutes before being strained and consumed. Tinctures are prepared by steeping the herb in alcohol or vinegar to extract its active compounds.

Dosage: The appropriate dosage of chaparral can vary depending on the specific form and intended use. It's important to follow the recommended dosage on the product label or consult with a healthcare professional for personalized guidance.

How to Use: Chaparral tea or tincture is typically taken orally. It can also be applied topically to the skin for certain conditions. It's important to use chaparral products as directed and to discontinue use if any adverse effects occur.

Side Effects: Chaparral is generally considered safe for most people when used in moderate amounts. However, excessive intake or prolonged use may lead to liver toxicity or other adverse effects. It may also interact with certain medications or have adverse effects in individuals with certain health conditions. It's important to use chaparral under the guidance of a healthcare professional and to discontinue use if any adverse effects occur.

Cocolmeca:

Definition: Cocolmeca, also known as Smilax ornata or sarsaparilla, is a flowering vine native to Mexico and Central America. It has been used traditionally in Mexican and Central American folk medicine for its purported medicinal properties.

Ingredients: Cocolmeca contains various bioactive compounds, including saponins, flavonoids, and plant sterols. These compounds are believed to contribute to the herb's medicinal properties, including its potential as a diuretic, blood purifier, and anti-inflammatory agent.

How to Prepare: Cocolmeca is commonly prepared and consumed as an herbal tea or decoction. To make tea, dried cocolmeca roots or leaves are steeped in hot water for several minutes before being strained and consumed. Decoctions involve boiling the roots or leaves in water to extract their active compounds.

Dosage: The appropriate dosage of cocolmeca can vary depending on factors such as age, health status, and the specific preparation being used. It's important to follow the recommended dosage on the product label or consult with a qualified herbalist or healthcare professional for personalized guidance.

How to Use: Cocolmeca tea or decoction is typically taken orally. It can also be used topically for certain skin conditions. It's important to use cocolmeca products as directed and to discontinue use if any adverse effects occur.

Side Effects: Cocolmeca is generally considered safe for most people when used in moderate amounts. However, excessive intake may lead to digestive upset or other adverse effects. It may also interact with certain medications or have adverse effects in individuals with certain health conditions. It's important to use cocolmeca under the guidance of a healthcare professional and to discontinue use if any adverse effects occur.

Contribo:

Definition: Contribo, also known as Aristolochiatrilobata, is a vine native to the Caribbean and Central America. It has been used traditionally in folk medicine for various purposes, including as a remedy for digestive issues, inflammation, and pain relief.

Ingredients: Contribo contains several bioactive compounds, including aristolochic acids, flavonoids, and alkaloids. These compounds are believed to contribute to the herb's medicinal properties, including its potential as an anti-inflammatory and analgesic agent.

How to Prepare: Contribo is typically prepared and consumed as an herbal tea or decoction. To make tea, dried contribo leaves or stems are steeped in hot water for several minutes before being strained and consumed. Decoctions involve boiling the leaves or stems in water to extract their active compounds.

Dosage: The appropriate dosage of contribo can vary depending on factors such as age, health status, and the specific preparation being used. It's important to follow the recommended dosage on the product label or consult with a qualified herbalist or healthcare professional for personalized guidance.

How to Use: Contribo tea or decoction is typically taken orally. It's important to use contribo products as directed and to discontinue use if any adverse effects occur.

Side Effects: Contribo contains aristolochic acids, which have been associated with serious adverse effects, including kidney damage and cancer. Due to these safety concerns, the use of contribo is highly discouraged, and it's important to avoid products containing aristolochic acids. Individuals should seek alternative remedies for their health needs.

Dandelion Root:

Definition: Dandelion, scientifically known as Taraxacum officinale, is a common flowering plant found worldwide. While often considered a pesky weed, dandelion has a long history of use in traditional medicine for its various health benefits.

Ingredients: Dandelion root contains several bioactive compounds, including sesquiterpene lactones, triterpenes, flavonoids, and polysaccharides. These compounds are believed to contribute to the herb's medicinal properties, including its potential as a diuretic, digestive aid, and liver tonic.

How to Prepare: Dandelion root can be prepared and consumed in various forms, including teas, tinctures, capsules, and extracts. To make tea, dried dandelion root is steeped in hot water for several minutes before being strained and consumed. Tinctures are prepared by steeping the root in alcohol or vinegar to extract its active compounds.

Dosage: The appropriate dosage of dandelion root can vary depending on factors such as age, health status, and the specific preparation being used. It's important to follow the recommended dosage on the product label or consult with a qualified herbalist or healthcare professional for personalized guidance.

How to Use: Dandelion root tea, tincture, or capsules are typically taken orally. It's important to use dandelion root products as directed and to discontinue use if any adverse effects occur.

Side Effects: Dandelion root is generally considered safe for most people when used in moderate amounts. However, some individuals may experience allergic reactions or digestive upset. It may also interact with certain medications or have adverse effects in individuals with certain health conditions. It's important to use dandelion root under the guidance of a healthcare professional and to discontinue use if any adverse effects occur.

Green Food Plus:

Definition: Green Food Plus is a dietary supplement formulated to provide a concentrated source of nutrients derived from various green plants. It's designed to support overall health and well-being by delivering essential vitamins, minerals, antioxidants, and phytonutrients.

Ingredients: Green Food Plus typically contains a blend of powdered green vegetables, grasses, algae, and other plant-based ingredients. Common ingredients may include wheatgrass, barley grass, spirulina, chlorella, alfalfa, kale, spinach, and broccoli, among others.

How to Prepare: Green Food Plus is usually available in powder form and can be mixed with water, juice, or smoothies. It's important to follow the recommended dosage on the product label and to consume it as part of a balanced diet.

Dosage: The appropriate dosage of Green Food Plus can vary depending on the specific product and individual needs. It's important to follow the recommended dosage on the product label or consult with a healthcare professional for personalized guidance.

How to Use: Green Food Plus powder is typically mixed with water, juice, or smoothies and consumed orally. It's often taken once or twice daily, preferably with meals, to maximize nutrient absorption.

Side Effects: Green Food Plus is generally considered safe for most people when used as directed. However, some individuals may experience digestive upset or allergic reactions to certain ingredients. It's important to consult with a healthcare provider before starting any new supplement regimen, especially if you have underlying health conditions or are taking medications.

Guaco:

Definition: Guaco, also known as Mikania cordata or Mikania glomerata, is a medicinal plant native to Central and South America. It has a long history of use in traditional medicine for its potential therapeutic properties.

Ingredients: Guaco contains several bioactive compounds, including coumarins, flavonoids, tannins, and saponins. These compounds are believed to contribute to the herb's medicinal properties, including its potential as an expectorant, anti-inflammatory, and antispasmodic agent.

How to Prepare: Guaco is typically prepared and consumed as an herbal tea or infusion. To make tea, dried guaco leaves are steeped in hot water for several minutes before being strained and consumed.

Dosage: The appropriate dosage of guaco can vary depending on factors such as age, health status, and the specific preparation being used. It's important to follow the recommended dosage on the product label or consult with a qualified herbalist or healthcare professional for personalized guidance.

How to Use: Guaco tea is typically taken orally. It can be consumed on its own or mixed with honey or other herbal teas for added flavor.

Side Effects: Guaco is generally considered safe for most people when used in moderate amounts. However, some individuals may experience allergic reactions or digestive upset. It may also interact with certain medications or have adverse effects in individuals with certain health conditions. It's important to use guaco under the guidance of a healthcare professional and to discontinue use if any adverse effects occur.

Irish Sea Moss:

Definition: Irish Sea Moss is a term often used interchangeably with Irish Moss, referring to the same species of red algae, Chondrus crispus. It's harvested from the rocky shores of the Atlantic coastlines of Europe and North America.

Ingredients: Irish Sea Moss shares the same nutritional profile as Irish Moss, containing iodine, vitamins, minerals, and polysaccharides. It's valued for its potential health benefits, including supporting thyroid function, boosting immune health, and promoting digestion.

How to Prepare: Irish Sea Moss is prepared in the same way as Irish Moss, by soaking it in water to rehydrate and soften it before use. It can be used in culinary applications or consumed as a dietary supplement.

Dosage: The dosage of Irish Sea Moss depends on the form and intended use. As a dietary supplement, it's important to follow the recommended dosage on the product label or consult with a healthcare professional for personalized guidance.

How to Use: Irish Sea Moss can be used in various culinary applications, including soups, smoothies, desserts, and sauces. It can also be consumed as a dietary supplement in the form of capsules, powders, or extracts.

Side Effects: Similar to Irish Moss, Irish Sea Moss is generally considered safe for most people when consumed in moderate amounts. However, individuals with seaweed allergies or sensitivities to carrageenan should exercise caution. It's important to discontinue use if any adverse effects occur and to consult with a healthcare professional if you have any concerns.

Lymphalin:

Definition: Lymphalin is a herbal supplement formulated to support lymphatic system health. The lymphatic system plays a crucial role in immune function and waste removal in the body, and Lymphalin is designed to promote its proper function.

Ingredients: Lymphalin typically contains a blend of herbs and botanical extracts known for their traditional use in supporting lymphatic system health. Common ingredients may include cleavers, red clover, echinacea, burdock root, and calendula, among others.

How to Prepare: Lymphalin is usually available in capsule or liquid form. Capsules are taken orally with water, while liquid forms may be mixed with water or juice before consumption. It's important to follow the recommended dosage on the product label.

Dosage: The appropriate dosage of Lymphalin can vary depending on the specific product and individual needs. It's important to follow the recommended dosage on the product label or consult with a healthcare professional for personalized guidance.

How to Use: Lymphalin capsules are typically taken orally with water, while liquid forms may be mixed with water or juice before consumption. It's often recommended to take Lymphalin on an empty stomach for optimal absorption.

Side Effects: Lymphalin is generally considered safe for most people when used as directed. However, some individuals may experience mild side effects such as gastrointestinal discomfort or allergic reactions to certain ingredients. It's important to consult with a healthcare provider before starting any new supplement regimen, especially if you have underlying health conditions or are taking medications.

Manjakani:

Definition: Manjakani, also known as Quercus infectoria or oak gall, is a natural substance derived from the oak tree. It has been used for centuries in traditional medicine for its potential health benefits, particularly for women's health and vaginal tightening.

Ingredients: Manjakani contains various bioactive compounds, including tannins, flavonoids, and gallic acid. These compounds are believed to contribute to the herb's medicinal properties, including its potential as an astringent and antiseptic agent.

How to Prepare: Manjakani is typically available in powder, capsule, or liquid extract form. It can be taken orally or used topically depending on the intended use. For vaginal tightening, manjakani may be applied topically as a gel or inserted into the vagina in capsule form.

Dosage: The appropriate dosage of manjakani can vary depending on factors such as age, health status, and the specific preparation being used. It's important to follow the recommended dosage on the product label or consult with a qualified herbalist or healthcare professional for personalized guidance.

How to Use: Manjakani can be taken orally or used topically depending on the intended use. It's important to use manjakani products as directed and to discontinue use if any adverse effects occur.

Side Effects: Manjakani is generally considered safe for most people when used in moderate amounts. However, some individuals may experience allergic reactions or skin irritation when used topically. It's important to use manjakani under the guidance of a healthcare professional and to discontinue use if any adverse effects occur.

Rhubarb:

Definition: Rhubarb, scientifically known as Rheum rhabarbarum, is a perennial plant cultivated for its edible stalks. While primarily used in culinary applications, rhubarb has also been utilized in traditional medicine for its potential health benefits, particularly for digestive health.

Ingredients: Rhubarb stalks contain various bioactive compounds, including anthraquinones (such as emodin and rhein), fiber, vitamins (such as vitamin K), and minerals (including calcium and potassium). These compounds are believed to contribute to the herb's medicinal properties, including its potential as a laxative and digestive aid.

How to Prepare: Rhubarb stalks are typically cooked before consumption, as the raw stalks are very tart and can be unpleasant to eat. They are often used in pies, crisps, jams, sauces, and other desserts, as well as in savory dishes. Rhubarb can also be used to make compotes, jams, and preserves.

Dosage: There is no specific dosage for rhubarb in culinary applications, as it is used as a food rather than a medicinal herb. However, when used for its potential laxative effects, it's important to consume rhubarb in moderation to avoid gastrointestinal upset.

How to Use: Rhubarb stalks can be chopped and cooked in various dishes, including pies, sauces, and jams. It's important to remove and discard the leaves, as they contain toxic compounds. When using rhubarb for its potential laxative effects, it's typically consumed as part of a cooked dish or in the form of a rhubarb-based herbal remedy.

Side Effects: Rhubarb stalks are generally safe for most people when consumed in moderate amounts as part of a balanced diet. However, excessive intake may lead to digestive upset or adverse effects due to the presence of oxalic acid, which can bind to calcium and form kidney stones in susceptible individuals. It's important to use rhubarb in moderation and to consult with a healthcare professional if you have any concerns or underlying health conditions.

Sarsaparilla:

Definition: Sarsaparilla refers to several species of plants belonging to the Smilax genus, including Smilax regelii and Smilax officinalis. It has been used historically in traditional medicine for its potential health benefits, particularly for its purported detoxifying and anti-inflammatory properties.

Ingredients: Sarsaparilla contains various bioactive compounds, including saponins (such as sarsaponin and smilagenin), flavonoids, phenolic acids, and sterols. These compounds are believed to contribute to the herb's medicinal properties, including its potential as a diuretic, blood purifier, and anti-inflammatory agent.

How to Prepare: Sarsaparilla root is typically prepared and consumed as an herbal tea, decoction, or tincture. To make tea, dried sarsaparilla root is steeped in hot water for several minutes before being strained and consumed. Decoctions involve boiling the root in water to extract its active compounds, while tinctures are prepared by steeping the root in alcohol or vinegar.

Dosage: The appropriate dosage of sarsaparilla can vary depending on factors such as age, health status, and the specific preparation being used. It's important to follow the recommended dosage on the product label or consult with a qualified herbalist or healthcare professional for personalized guidance.

How to Use: Sarsaparilla tea or tincture is typically taken orally. It's important to use sarsaparilla products as directed and to discontinue use if any adverse effects occur.

Side Effects: Sarsaparilla is generally considered safe for most people when used in moderate amounts. However, some individuals may experience allergic reactions or digestive upset. It may also interact with certain medications or have adverse effects in individuals with certain health conditions. It's important to use sarsaparilla under the guidance of a healthcare professional and to discontinue use if any adverse effects occur.

Tila:

Definition: Tila, also known as linden flower or lime blossom, refers to the flowers of the Tilia genus, primarily Tilia europaea and Tilia cordata. These trees are native to Europe, but they are also cultivated in other regions for their fragrant and medicinal flowers.

Ingredients: Tila flowers contain various bioactive compounds, including flavonoids, phenolic acids, and volatile oils. These compounds are believed to contribute to the herb's medicinal properties, including its potential as a mild sedative, anxiolytic, and anti-inflammatory agent.

How to Prepare: Tila flowers are typically prepared and consumed as an herbal tea or infusion. To make tea, dried tila flowers are steeped in hot water for several minutes before being strained and consumed.

Dosage: The appropriate dosage of tila can vary depending on factors such as age, health status, and the specific preparation being used. It's important to follow the recommended dosage on the product label or consult with a qualified herbalist or healthcare professional for personalized guidance.

How to Use: Tila tea is typically taken orally. It's often consumed in the evening as a calming bedtime beverage or during times of stress or anxiety. It's important to use tila products as directed and to discontinue use if any adverse effects occur.

Side Effects: Tila is generally considered safe for most people when used in moderate amounts. However, some individuals may experience allergic reactions or digestive upset. It may also interact with certain medications or have adverse effects in individuals with certain health conditions. It's important to use tila under the guidance of a healthcare professional and to discontinue use if any adverse effects occur.

Valerian:

Definition: Valerian, scientifically known as Valeriana officinalis, is a perennial flowering plant native to Europe and Asia. It has been used for centuries in traditional medicine for its potential calming and sedative effects.

Ingredients: Valerian root contains several bioactive compounds, including valerenic acid, valepotriates, and volatile oils. These compounds are believed to contribute to the herb's medicinal properties, including its potential as a sedative, anxiolytic, and sleep aid.

How to Prepare: Valerian root is typically prepared and consumed as an herbal tea, tincture, or capsule. To make tea, dried valerian root is steeped in hot water for several minutes before being strained and consumed. Tinctures are prepared by steeping the root in alcohol or vinegar to extract its active compounds.

Dosage: The appropriate dosage of valerian can vary depending on factors such as age, health status, and the specific preparation being used. It's important to follow the recommended dosage on the product label or consult with a qualified herbalist or healthcare professional for personalized guidance.

How to Use: Valerian tea, tincture, or capsules are typically taken orally. It's often consumed in the evening as a sleep aid or during times of stress or anxiety. It's important to use valerian products as directed and to discontinue use if any adverse effects occur.

Side Effects: Valerian is generally considered safe for most people when used in moderate amounts. However, some individuals may experience mild side effects such as drowsiness, headache, or gastrointestinal upset. It may also interact with certain medications or have adverse effects in individuals with certain health conditions. It's important to use valerian under the guidance of a healthcare professional and to discontinue use if any adverse effects occur.

Wild Cherry Bark:

Definition: Wild cherry bark, scientifically known as Prunus serotina, is the bark obtained from the black cherry tree native to North America. It has been used traditionally in Native American and folk medicine for its potential health benefits, particularly for respiratory and digestive issues.

Ingredients: Wild cherry bark contains various bioactive compounds, including cyanogenic glycosides (such as prunasin and amygdalin), flavonoids, and phenolic acids. These compounds are believed to contribute to the herb's medicinal properties, including its potential as an expectorant, cough suppressant, and mild sedative.

How to Prepare: Wild cherry bark is typically prepared and consumed as an herbal tea, decoction, or syrup. To make tea, dried wild cherry bark is steeped in hot water for several minutes before being strained and consumed. Decoctions involve boiling the bark in water to extract its active compounds, while syrups are made by simmering the bark with sugar or honey to create a thick, sweet liquid.

Dosage: The appropriate dosage of wild cherry bark can vary depending on factors such as age, health status, and the specific preparation being used. It's important to follow the recommended dosage on the product label or consult with a qualified herbalist or healthcare professional for personalized guidance.

How to Use: Wild cherry bark tea, decoction, or syrup is typically taken orally. It's often consumed to soothe coughs, sore throats, and other respiratory symptoms. It's important to use wild cherry bark products as directed and to discontinue use if any adverse effects occur.

Side Effects: Wild cherry bark is generally considered safe for most people when used in moderate amounts. However, it contains cyanogenic glycosides, which can release cyanide in the body when metabolized. While the risk of cyanide poisoning from consuming wild cherry bark is low when used appropriately, excessive intake or prolonged use may lead to adverse effects. It's important to use wild cherry bark under the guidance of a healthcare professional and to discontinue use if any adverse effects occur.

Yellowdock:

Definition: Yellowdock, scientifically known as Rumex crispus, is a perennial flowering plant native to Europe and western Asia but is also found in North America. It has a long history of use in traditional medicine, particularly among Indigenous peoples, for its potential health benefits.

Ingredients: Yellowdock root contains various bioactive compounds, including anthraquinone glycosides (such as emodin and chrysophanol), tannins, and vitamins (including vitamin A and vitamin C). These compounds are believed to contribute to the herb's medicinal properties, including its potential as a laxative, blood cleanser, and liver tonic.

How to Prepare: Yellowdock root is typically prepared and consumed as an herbal tea, tincture, or capsule. To make tea, dried yellowdock root is steeped in hot water for several minutes before being strained and consumed. Tinctures are prepared by steeping the root in alcohol or vinegar to extract its active compounds.

Dosage: The appropriate dosage of yellowdock can vary depending on factors such as age, health status, and the specific preparation being used. It's important to follow the recommended dosage on the product label or consult with a qualified herbalist or healthcare professional for personalized guidance.

How to Use: Yellowdock tea, tincture, or capsules are typically taken orally. It's often consumed to support digestion, promote bowel regularity, and cleanse the blood. It's important to use yellowdock products as directed and to discontinue use if any adverse effects occur.

Side Effects: Yellowdock is generally considered safe for most people when used in moderate amounts. However, some individuals may experience mild side effects such as gastrointestinal upset or allergic reactions. It may also interact with certain medications or have adverse effects in individuals with certain health conditions. It's important to use yellowdock under the guidance of a healthcare professional and to discontinue use if any adverse effects occur.

Yellowdock Root:

Definition: Yellowdock root, scientifically known as Rumex crispus, is the root of a perennial flowering plant native to Europe and western Asia, also found in North America. It has a long history of use in traditional medicine, particularly among Indigenous peoples, for its potential health benefits.

Ingredients: Yellowdock root contains various bioactive compounds, including anthraquinone glycosides (such as emodin and chrysophanol), tannins, and vitamins (including vitamin A and vitamin C). These compounds are believed to contribute to the herb's medicinal properties, including its potential as a laxative, blood cleanser, and liver tonic.

How to Prepare: Yellowdock root is typically prepared and consumed as an herbal tea, tincture, or capsule. To make tea, dried yellowdock root is steeped in hot water for several minutes before being strained and consumed. Tinctures are prepared by steeping the root in alcohol or vinegar to extract its active compounds.

Dosage: The appropriate dosage of yellowdock root can vary depending on factors such as age, health status, and the specific preparation being used. It's important to follow the recommended dosage on the product label or consult with a qualified herbalist or healthcare professional for personalized guidance.

How to Use: Yellowdock root tea, tincture, or capsules are typically taken orally. It's often consumed to support digestion, promote bowel regularity, and cleanse the blood. It's important to use yellowdock root products as directed and to discontinue use if any adverse effects occur.

Side Effects: Yellowdock root is generally considered safe for most people when used in moderate amounts. However, some individuals may experience mild side effects such as gastrointestinal upset or allergic reactions. It may also interact with certain medications or have adverse effects in individuals with certain health conditions. It's important to use yellowdock root under the guidance of a healthcare professional and to discontinue use if any adverse effects occur.

Agrimony:

Definition: Agrimony, scientifically known as Agrimonia eupatoria, is a perennial herbaceous plant native to Europe, Asia, and North America. It has a long history of use in traditional medicine, particularly in European folk medicine, for its potential health benefits.

Ingredients: Agrimony contains various bioactive compounds, including tannins, flavonoids, phenolic acids, and volatile oils. These compounds are believed to contribute to the herb's medicinal properties, including its potential as an astringent, anti-inflammatory, and digestive aid.

How to Prepare: Agrimony is typically prepared and consumed as an herbal tea, tincture, or poultice. To make tea, dried agrimony leaves and flowers are steeped in hot water for several minutes before being strained and consumed. Tinctures are prepared by steeping the herb in alcohol or vinegar to extract its active compounds.

Dosage: The appropriate dosage of agrimony can vary depending on factors such as age, health status, and the specific preparation being used. It's important to follow the recommended dosage on the product label or consult with a qualified herbalist or healthcare professional for personalized guidance.

How to Use: Agrimony tea, tincture, or poultice is typically taken orally or applied topically. It's often consumed to soothe gastrointestinal issues, such as indigestion and diarrhea, or used externally to treat skin conditions.

Side Effects: Agrimony is generally considered safe for most people when used in moderate amounts. However, some individuals may experience allergic reactions or gastrointestinal upset. It may also interact with certain medications or have adverse effects in individuals with certain health conditions. It's important to use agrimony under the guidance of a healthcare professional and to discontinue use if any adverse effects occur.

Alfalfa:

Definition: Alfalfa, scientifically known as Medicago sativa, is a flowering plant in the pea family native to Asia but cultivated worldwide. It's primarily grown as fodder for livestock, but it has also been used in traditional medicine for its potential health benefits.

Ingredients: Alfalfa contains various bioactive compounds, including vitamins (such as vitamin A, vitamin C, and vitamin K), minerals (including calcium, magnesium, and potassium), amino acids, and phytoestrogens. These compounds are believed to contribute to the herb's medicinal properties, including its potential as a nutritive tonic, diuretic, and hormone balancer.

How to Prepare: Alfalfa is typically consumed as sprouts, herbal tea, or in supplement form (such as capsules or tablets). To make tea, dried alfalfa leaves are steeped in hot water for several minutes before being strained and consumed.

Dosage: The appropriate dosage of alfalfa can vary depending on factors such as age, health status, and the specific preparation being used. It's important to follow the recommended dosage on the product label or consult with a qualified herbalist or healthcare professional for personalized guidance.

How to Use: Alfalfa sprouts, tea, or supplements are typically taken orally. It's often consumed as a dietary supplement to support overall health and well-being, as well as to promote kidney health and hormone balance.

Side Effects: Alfalfa is generally considered safe for most people when consumed in moderate amounts. However, some individuals may experience allergic reactions or digestive upset. It may also interact with certain medications or have adverse effects in individuals with certain health conditions, such as autoimmune diseases or hormone-sensitive conditions. Pregnant or breastfeeding individuals should consult with a healthcare professional before using alfalfa supplements. It's important to use alfalfa under the guidance of a healthcare professional and to discontinue use if any adverse effects occur.

Ashwagandha:

Definition: Ashwagandha, scientifically known as Withaniasomnifera, is a small shrub native to India, the Middle East, and parts of Africa. It has a long history of use in Ayurvedic medicine for its potential health benefits, particularly for its adaptogenic properties.

Ingredients: Ashwagandha root contains various bioactive compounds, including alkaloids (such as withanolides), steroidal lactones, and flavonoids. These compounds are believed to contribute to the herb's medicinal properties, including its potential as an adaptogen, anti-inflammatory, and immune-modulating agent.

How to Prepare: Ashwagandha is typically consumed as a powdered root, herbal tea, tincture, or in supplement form (such as capsules or tablets). To make tea, dried ashwagandha root is steeped in hot water for several minutes before being strained and consumed.

Dosage: The appropriate dosage of ashwagandha can vary depending on factors such as age, health status, and the specific preparation being used. It's important to follow the recommended dosage on the product label or consult with a qualified herbalist or healthcare professional for personalized guidance.

How to Use: Ashwagandha powder, tea, tincture, or supplements are typically taken orally. It's often consumed to support stress management, promote relaxation, and boost overall vitality and well-being.

Side Effects: Ashwagandha is generally considered safe for most people when used in moderate amounts. However, some individuals may experience mild side effects such as gastrointestinal upset or drowsiness. It may also interact with certain medications or have adverse effects in individuals with certain health conditions, such as autoimmune diseases or thyroid disorders. Pregnant or breastfeeding individuals should consult with a healthcare professional before using ashwagandha supplements. It's important to use ashwagandha under the guidance of a healthcare professional and to discontinue use if any adverse effects occur.

Irish Moss:

Definition: Irish Moss, scientifically known as Chondrus crispus, is a species of red algae or seaweed native to the Atlantic coastlines of Europe and North America. It has been used for centuries in traditional Irish and Scottish cuisine, as well as in herbal medicine.

Ingredients: Irish Moss is rich in various nutrients, including iodine, sulfur compounds, vitamins (such as vitamin A, vitamin K, and vitamin B12), minerals (including calcium, magnesium, potassium, and sodium), and polysaccharides (such as carrageenan). These nutrients are believed to contribute to the herb's potential health benefits.

How to Prepare: Irish Moss is typically prepared by soaking it in water to rehydrate and soften it before use. It can be added to soups, stews, smoothies, desserts, and other dishes as a thickening agent or nutritional supplement.

Dosage: The appropriate dosage of Irish Moss can vary depending on factors such as age, health status, and the specific preparation being used. It's important to follow recipes or guidelines for culinary use and to consult with a healthcare professional for guidance on using Irish Moss as a dietary supplement.

How to Use: Irish Moss can be used in culinary applications to add thickness and nutritional value to dishes. It can also be consumed as a dietary supplement in the form of capsules, powders, or extracts.

Side Effects: Irish Moss is generally considered safe for most people when consumed in moderate amounts as part of a balanced diet. However, some individuals may be allergic to seaweed or carrageenan, a compound found in Irish Moss that is used as a food additive. It's important to discontinue use if any adverse effects occur and to consult with a healthcare professional if you have any concerns.

Burdock:

Definition: Burdock, scientifically known as Arctium lappa, is a biennial plant native to Europe and Asia but now found worldwide. It's part of the Asteraceae family and has been used for centuries in traditional medicine and culinary practices.

Ingredients: Burdock contains various nutrients, including carbohydrates, fiber, vitamins (such as vitamin B6, folate, and vitamin C), and minerals (including potassium, magnesium, and manganese). It also contains active compounds such as polyphenols and volatile oils.

How to Prepare: Burdock can be prepared and consumed in various ways. The roots, leaves, and seeds are all utilized for different purposes. The root is commonly used in cooking, herbal teas, tinctures, and supplements, while the leaves and seeds are sometimes used in herbal preparations.

Dosage: The appropriate dosage of burdock root can vary depending on the specific form and intended use. For culinary purposes, there are no strict dosage guidelines, but for supplements or herbal remedies, it's essential to follow the recommended dosage on the product label or consult with a healthcare professional.

How to Use: Burdock root can be used in cooking by peeling, slicing, and adding it to soups, stews, stir-fries, or salads. It can also be brewed into a tea or used to make tinctures or extracts for medicinal purposes. Some people may also take burdock root supplements in capsule or powder form.

Side Effects: While burdock is generally considered safe for most people when consumed in moderate amounts, some individuals may experience allergic reactions or digestive upset. Additionally, burdock may interact with certain medications or have adverse effects in individuals with certain health conditions, such as diabetes or allergies to plants in the Asteraceae family. It's important to consult with a healthcare provider before using burdock, especially if you have underlying health conditions or are taking medications.

Cascara Sagrada:

Definition: Cascara Sagrada, scientifically known as Rhamnus purshiana, is a species of buckthorn native to western North America. It has been used traditionally as a laxative and to promote bowel regularity.

Ingredients: The primary active ingredients in cascara sagrada are anthraquinone glycosides, particularly cascarosides A and B. These compounds stimulate peristalsis in the colon, leading to increased bowel movements.

How to Prepare: Cascara sagrada is typically prepared as an herbal tea, tincture, or capsule. To make tea, dried cascara sagrada bark is steeped in hot water for several minutes before being strained and consumed. Tinctures are prepared by steeping the bark in alcohol to extract its active compounds.

Dosage: The appropriate dosage of cascara sagrada can vary depending on the specific preparation and intended use. It's important to follow the recommended dosage on the product label or consult with a healthcare professional for personalized guidance.

How to Use: Cascara sagrada tea or tincture is typically taken orally. It's important to start with a low dose and gradually increase if needed to avoid potential side effects such as cramping or diarrhea.

Side Effects: Cascara sagrada is considered safe for short-term use when used as directed. However, long-term or excessive use may lead to dependence, electrolyte imbalance, or dehydration. It may also interact with certain medications or have adverse effects in individuals with certain health conditions. It's important to use cascara sagrada under the guidance of a healthcare professional and to discontinue use if any adverse effects occur.

THE END

www.ingramcontent.com/pod-product-compliance
Lightning Source LLC
Chambersburg PA
CBHW081557250726
48653CB00009B/3469